MW00425711

The Survival Guide

For

Nursing Students

By Janelle Garrett

Edited by Sheree Phillips

Cover Design by Poole Publishing

For Mom and Dad

Whatever venture I want to take, you support me.

It means the world.

Thank you

A special thanks to Kim, Nicole, and Nerissa for your help and thoughts. You guys are the real heroes. Saving lives by day, editing manuscripts by night. You are the type of nurses that deserve awards. Thanks to my students who I precepted. You make some dang good caregivers, and sparked the idea for this guide.

Prologue

I stood before a closed door on the 7th Tower of a busy, bustling hospital in downtown Orlando. Although my stethoscope hung proudly around my neck, I wished for a brief moment that it would come to life and strangle me before I walked inside the room. It was my first day on an actual nursing unit as a student, and my stomach cramped so badly I thought I would throw up.

A dozen thoughts raced through my head.

How did I get here? Will the nurse I'm working with eat me, like all the stories? Everyone knows nurses are ogres when it came to students, chewing them up and then spitting them back out again to run home after every clinical and cry themselves to sleep. Oh God, what if the patient is horrible? Will they even let me do an assessment? Some patients don't like new students, because clearly we don't know what we are doing. If they don't let me do any assessment, I won't pass clinicals. I'll be kicked out of the program and there goes two years of my life for nothing.

WHAT IF THE PATIENT DIES?

Welcome to the inner thoughts of every single student about to meet their first patient. Unbeknownst to me at the time, of course. I thought I was the only one freaking out, and wished I could be like those confident "cool" kids that exist even in college. You know the ones. The students who breeze into a patient's room acting like they own the place, whip through an assessment like a seasoned nurse, and laugh all the way to straight A's.

Well, if you're like myself and the other 99% of nursing students, this guide is for you. And this guide is also for those "cool" students, because I suspect that deep inside you're scared, too. At some point every nursing student will lose sleep over nerves in your first semester. You might throw up. You might pass out at the first sight of blood. You might think of quitting before you even start.

Take my advice, okay? I've been there. In fact, for the first several weeks I was *perpetually* there. During every single clinical I thought I was going to die from nerves. And there is still that little voice in my head that says, "I'm not good enough, smart enough, compassionate enough...in fact, I will fail."

Let's do an exercise together. Ready?

Silence that voice once and for all. Trust me. You'll feel better.

The reality is that even the most seasoned nurse stood in your shoes at one time. Every single one. From the CNO of the metropolitan hospital to the ER nurse saving lives or putting bandaids on a scrape, to the OR nurse recognizing signs of allergic reactions to anesthesia or having to put up with the surgeon's dumb jokes...they stood in your shoes.

I pushed through the door into the patient's room that day. The guy didn't even wake up, but slept as the

2

nurse and I checked on him. I was relieved when I didn't have to touch him and we left to come back later. Then the second time I pushed through the door it was just a little easier. And the third time was easier than the second, until one day, the nerves were less and the confidence was more. So goes the story for everyone, and so too, will be *your* story.

Take a deep breath, my friend. You got this.

Chapter 1 – Before You Even Start School

Do you have what it takes to be a nurse? That's a question you probably (or at least *should)* have asked yourself. It's more than just pure competency, more than the ability to think on your feet, go nose to nose with death and not blink first, or be able to hold a crying family member as they go through a horrible, unexpected diagnosis. Competency, although important, is not the only consideration.

What is, then? Let's talk about three important considerations before you even start nursing school.

The Myth of Not Having a Life

Let me just set the record straight: you *can* have a life outside of nursing school. Please, for the sake of your sanity, do not believe the lies you've heard or told yourself. Perhaps it was well intentioned. Maybe you have geared yourself up for not socializing for four years. Or maybe you've decided to put off marriage, traveling, or kids for the sake of school. I'll be honest: that might be a good idea for some people. But is that a good idea for you?

It's not an either/or situation. That is a fallacy, one that students often fall into. Either I have to commit 100% to nursing school, or I shouldn't go. Granted, nursing school is not for the faint of heart. You will pull your hair out over tests, have nightmares about those mean floor nurses and techs who hate you, and cry to your teacher asking for an extension on an assignment. But allow me to stand on a soap box for a minute.

You are a human being with dignity, worth, and needs. That means you need balance in your life; the ability to be free to explore who you are as a person outside of the crushing expectations you and others place on nursing students. It is possible to balance school, work, family, leisure, and spiritual needs. In fact, it's vital that you are able to do these things. Otherwise, you will burn out. And I don't mean in a few years after graduation. You will burn out *in school,* by quitting, hating your life, or being bitter once you graduate.

I was lucky enough to have already come to grips with this before school. I watched as student after student in my class either dropped out in the first semester, or *lost their minds* over tests and clinicals. Some became walking zombies or hysterical messes, or wrongly relied on their personalities rather than embracing the sheer hard work nursing school requires. Several times I was asked to help my suffering fellow students complete their paperwork during clinicals or hug them while they cried in a cubby somewhere. I was a B student. I'll just say that outright. But being a B student who had a firm grasp on who I was as a person, what I was capable of or not capable of, and not ignoring my friends and family, was worth it to me.

You will have to make that decision. Maybe A's will come easy to you. If so, I'm jealous and you should thank your lucky stars. But if not, you will be faced with that question: will you maintain a healthy and balanced life outside of school, or will you sacrifice it on the altar of the ever-elusive 4.0 GPA? I'll let you into a secret. I've interviewed people and didn't take a single glance at their GPA. What was important to me was are they well-rounded, articulate, and passionate about what they were pursuing? That had nothing to do with whether they got an A in Pharmacology or not.

The Truth of Body/Mind/Spirit Balance

Don't skip this section. I can already see you overachievers skimming over this, scoffing at the mumbo-jumbo you think is coming. Do so to your own peril. Okay, maybe that was a bit dramatic.

I'm not going to build an argument for the belief that we are persons with three distinct essences. I will assume most of you are educated enough to have a general idea of what I mean. What I *do* want to build an argument for is that understanding how these three things play a role in your personal life will only benefit you as you are in school. As a nurse, you will learn that caring for patient's physical needs must also be combined with caring for their psychological, emotional and spiritual needs. We must see the whole body person, not just the physical. And this is true for you, as well.

You can only help another person to the degree that you can help yourself. Who are you? Really. Deep down. The core of you. What are your physical needs? Food. Water. Health. Are you tending to those? If you aren't, how can you expect to tend to the physical needs of others?

What are your emotional and mental needs? Perhaps you battle anxiety, depression, OCD, or a host of other mental or emotional struggles. Are you tending to those? If not, you will cycle through nursing school just like you cycle through other aspects of your life. Having a good grasp of these needs, and knowing how to care for yourself when they rear their heads, will only benefit you. If not, what will happen when depression hits and you're in the middle of finals?

What are your spiritual needs? This one can be a little tricky. I'm not going to advocate for one religion or spiritual experience over another. But whether we are monotheistic, atheist, or skeptic, we all have a spiritual aspect to our lives. These things must be tended to. Does prayer or meditation help you to keep calm amidst the turmoil of your personal life? Knowing how to stop, take a deep breath, take a break from studying, and get in tune with your spiritual self, will aid in this body/mind/spirit balance. Knowing who you are as a person and with these combined elements will help get you through not just stress, but also traumatic experiences that arise.

Here is what I mean.

It was my last semester. I was a senior nurse tech. This meant that I had certain privileges, like the ability to start IV's, get paid when I worked, and be groomed to land a good job after graduation. At this point I had seen it all: blood, vomit, feces, death...everything. During one shift the emergent bay was stirring as a patient was rushed in. I was working down the hall and peeked over to see what the deal was. The nurse I was working with passed by, so I asked her what had come in.

"A drug overdose," she said, looking back over her shoulder with compassion in her eyes. "A young kid."

Just then several family members came rushing in; I watched as a nurse took them aside to explain what was going on. The family collapsed into tears and sobs.

No one can prepare you for how this will impact you emotionally. We are all different. But for me it was heart-wrenching. I have a hard time, and still do, shutting off my emotions when I see suffering. To an extent, this is what separates a good nurse from a *great* nurse. But then the black hole hits. Every nurse knows what I mean. It's that point at which you have to decide whether you will snap or bend.

Have you ever seen the difference between bending a healthy stick or snapping a dead one? A healthy stick is malleable. It will eventually break when enough pressure is exerted, but first it will bend with that pressure. If the bending doesn't break it, it will snap back to where it was. However, a brittle stick will snap with far less pressure. It's dry and dead, and once its snapped it can't go back to what it used to be.

Seeing the suffering bent me. But it didn't break me. Why? Because I knew three things. First, I knew the patient was in good hands. A team of professionals was seeing to their physical needs. Second, I didn't cut myself completely off emotionally or psychologically. I embraced the empathy without letting it crush me. And third, I trusted that God knew what he was doing. My faith allowed me to push through the sorrow and acknowledge that sometimes things just don't make sense. God's plans are far above my own.

This process will look different for you. But if you don't understand your own Body/Mind/Spirit needs, you won't be able to appropriately balance your reactions when things don't go as expected. Maybe you will, like me, see incredible suffering. Or maybe you won't get the grade you needed. Perhaps a personal crisis will arise outside of the school setting, requiring that you tend to things at home. Whatever the case, embracing yourself and the unique way your whole person responds to environmental things outside your control will only help you. It's vital that you commit to this *before* the stressors of school make this all the more difficult.

Here is some down-to-earth, practical advice.

For your physical needs: Get into an exercise and eating routine. I gained twenty pounds in nursing school. I wish I had not neglected this important piece of my life. If you are already doing this, excellent, you are ahead of the curve. What you can do, though, is vow to not neglect your physical body for one of the other needs.

For your emotional and psychological needs: I have two recommendations. First, see a therapist or counselor. Yes, I'm serious. I'm a huge believer in this. All of us are flawed and broken in one way or another. Talking with someone can help you process through your own life story. If you prefer not to see a professional, find a trustworthy and wise friend who is also a good listener. Maybe a mentor from your church, synagogue, or temple. A pastor or priest. A person within your social circles that you admire and trust. Just choose a person whose own life is balanced, someone you can look at and say, "There are some things about this person I really admire." Talking is therapeutic for both introverts and extroverts. Second, don't be afraid to go on medication for mood disorders. See a doctor if you suspect you might need some. Together you can come up with a regimen that works for you.

For your spiritual needs: This one is tricky, because, well, it just is. Depending on your religion, get involved in that community. If you aren't religious, this doesn't mean you aren't spiritual. Find somewhere you are comfortable, accepted, and have a support system to help you. You don't have to believe in organized religion, or even believe in God, to still need the help of others. Since I'm the one writing this book and believe in God, I can say this. Religion brings a lot of comfort to a lot of people during times of stress and trial. Don't close yourself off from that resource should the time arise that you need it. In fact, it might be the very thing that draws you closer to God, and that God uses to show you that maybe, just maybe, there is something to be said about learning more about Him.

Chapter Two – Your First Semester

Congratulations. You've done as advised and have prepared yourself by not believing you can't have a life, and by embracing the way your Body/Mind/Spirit interact together to form who you are as a person. You've told your friends and family that you will still go out with them once in a while. You've assured your kids that you will still love them even when you are studying all night for a midterm. You've explained to your spouse that they will remain a priority even when your life gets crazy busy.

Now what?

I was pleasantly surprised when someone plopped a brand new laptop in front of me that first orientation day. True, I had paid for it. But still, I needed to learn how it worked. What programs there were and how to use them. Where the dang on and off button was so it could operate in the first place.

I wished someone had told me to chill out about all the practical stuff and get to know my professors and clinical instructors.

The Myth That You Should Take Criticism Personally

It's absolutely true that some teachers are just mean. But I can promise you with 99% certainty that an instructor's personality, lecturing skills, empathy or meanness is irrelevant. What matters is how committed you are to learning.

There will always be those teachers who intimidate even the brightest and the best. Do yourself a favor and try as hard as possible to be placed in their clinical group. Trust me on this one. There are several reasons for this. First, as a nurse you won't have much control over who your patients are. The more prepared you are for the moody and demanding ones, the better. I found that my most disliked instructors ended up being the ones who best prepared me for the real nursing world. This doesn't mean you sit back and let them verbally abuse you. What this does mean is that you need to learn how to do your job in the midst of it. Second, your teachers really do care about you, even the mean ones who tell you you're going to kill your patients or push your emotions to the brink. The reality is, they know what they are talking about. You really *could* kill someone. Your instructor doesn't go to bed at night scheming ways to shame you. They go to bed grateful that nobody died or made a horrible mistake. When they lecture you, it's because they care about you and the patient.

As an aside, the vast majority of instructors are awesome. So make a mental note not to freak out at
14

every new clinical assignment you get. And even on those days that you dread, there is always a lesson. That patient, or that instructor, has something valuable to teach you, good or bad. The good experiences we have can pop up in unexpected places. And the bad experiences are teachers. You will grow, expand, and learn how to cope in new ways, regardless.

The Myth That Arrogance is Confidence

For some reason, most people equate humility with weakness. The opposite, however, is true. It takes a strong person to realize they don't know everything. If you go into nursing school as an eager learner rather than to prove all you know, it will change your nursing experience. This is true after graduation, too. Just because you have "RN" behind your name doesn't make you a great nurse.

Humility isn't natural, it's learned. People fall into two basic categories: the victors and the defeated. There are those who beat their chests and subdue their enemies, and those who cower in the shadows and pray no one notices them.

The humble step into the light, not with a chip on their shoulder or a downcast eye, but with quiet strength that is ready for anything. When your instructor sees that, you will stand out. It will exude from you. You're the one who isn't afraid to ask a question when you're confused. The student who is the first to volunteer for something you've never done before. The fellow learner who is willing offer help to someone who is struggling even if you don't have all the answers.

My favorite students on the unit are always the ones who don't disappear, but stay by my side asking questions. The ones I care nothing about? They are the ones who are arrogant, never asking questions, follow and watch without saying a word, or talk about anything besides what they are learning. They are the ones who then disappear to get ahead on homework in the break room to maintain their GPA.

Humility doesn't mean you can't be strong in your opinion or have a go get 'em attitude. What it does mean is that your passion is first for the patient, and then for learning. If your priorities are in that order, I can guarantee that your instructor will be impressed.

The Myth That Nurses Eat Their Young

Now that you have the eye of your clinical instructor and teachers because you are ready to work and learn, what happens when you step onto the floor for the first time? Let's say it's a thirty bed unit on the cardiology floor. You are nervous yet confident. You are pretty sure you won't kill anyone. You like your fellow students and your instructor kind of scares you, but he or she seems to be happy they are a teacher. They don't hate their job.

Now what? This may seem like an unnecessary given but hear me out: You actually have to *talk* to your patients and the nurse you are assigned to.

We are not monsters. We are real people with families, pets, and friends. We like to eat food. We like to be able to pee every once in a while. We don't get along with everyone. We go to church. We yell and complain to refs at sporting events. We like going for drinks. We like reading at home, alone. We think the Hunger Games was awesome. We really, really hate olives. We stub our toes and curse. We snore when we sleep. We think Adam Sandler is funny, but that his movies are annoying. Frogs scare us.

You get where I'm going with that. We know you are people, too. We know you are scared out of your mind. We know you don't want to mess up. And for the vast majority of us, we don't really mind you are there unless you just sit there, do nothing and try to make everyone think you already know everything.

Just Do Something

As a nurse, I had a huge pet peeves. Want to know what it was for me, and probably the vast majority of other nurses? Students who sit and stare and don't do anything. They clog the halls. They talk in groups laughing.

They follow their instructor like ducklings and don't jump in and *do* something. They take two hour lunch breaks.

You will get what you put into the experience.

Now, safety first, my friends. Follow whatever rules and guidelines your school has set. But for the love of all things holy, *ask your nurse what you can do*. Ask them what they are doing and if you can do it, too, as long as it doesn't break protocol. If there is something cool and exciting going on with your patient and it's time to go to lunch...don't go to lunch. Tell your instructor a patient is getting a paracentesis and you want to watch. I promise they will say yes.

I LOVED teaching students. In fact, six months after I got my first job, I was asked to be a preceptor, often for two students at a time. It was by far my favorite job.

Guess which students I suggested get job interviews?

The ones who didn't disappear. The ones who asked me if I needed help even when everyone else was going on break. The ones who asked a million questions. Sure, you may be in your first semester, but do you want a job as a nurse tech? Or maybe you really loved Orthopedics (where I worked) and wanted me to put in a good word in a few semesters when you graduate. You can bet your last dime I did. And guess what? They got the interview, and often got the job. I had at least five or six students I precepted get jobs on my unit. Five or six. That shows you that the vast majority of students don't stand out. Your nurse has the ability to influence whether you get a hearing with a nurse manager or not. It's called networking, and it's a very, very valuable skill to have, even early on in the game. I promise that the paperwork you have to get done can wait. Don't sacrifice hands-on experience for a flawless clinical sheet.

Chapter Three – The Middle Semesters

You've survived your first semester. That's a huge accomplishment. Some statistics estimate that up to 60% of nursing students will drop out before graduation. Let's you and I decide right this minute that this won't be you! If you survived your first semester, you can make it all the way through.

I'm glad we got that out of the way. Now, on to the middle semesters. This is the time where you start to feel more confident but wow...no one told you how long the months are. Between school, your job, maybe your kids and marriage, your commitment to your friends and family, weddings, seeing a movie now and then, deaths in the family...things can pile up. What are your priorities?

The Myth of Dropping Out

Rumor has it that the first semester is the hardest. While this may be true for some, this isn't true for others. Not for me, anyway. The hardest semester for me was somewhere in the three to four range. It's where life is slogging, where you feel stuck in mud and studying is just downright hard. You've got some experience, sure, and the "baby love" has worn off. It's like having a one-year-old who won't sleep. That's the middle semesters. You have a puppy that's almost potty-trained but refuses to poop anywhere except the living room floor. This is where the rubber meets the road.

You've asked yourself a million times: do I have what it takes? Because from where you are standing, life just keeps happening and getting in the way of school. Grandma dies and you have to fly to the funeral. You get engaged and have to plan a wedding. Your son is graduating high school and you have to plan his party. You go through a divorce. You scratch your head and wonder...where can school fall in all this? Maybe you should find a cave somewhere to hide in until you're done. You can just have your spouse throw you food every once in a while, turn off all digital media so no one can find you, and only leave your room for clinicals. And maybe to shower every once in a while so your patients aren't repulsed.

Priorities Are Possible

This goes back to the first chapter, and this probably won't be the last time I mention it either. Back before you started nursing school you decided you would have a life. What you didn't know was that life would constantly be pulling you away from studying. Take my hand and remember this: You have worth and dignity. You are not defined by how tired you are, what your grades are, or whether your preceptor likes you.

As I have mentioned, I precepted quite often. The students who were in the middle semesters were the most tired. One of them was going through a divorce. One was getting married. One was considering moving. All of them had one thing in common: school was a burden.

Reality check: *nursing school is a burden*. Sure, it's fun. You learn a lot. You love what you do. But the weight will settle on you, and the decision before you will be whether you think you can handle it. Will you study your butt off for that A? Excellent. Sometimes that means you have to sacrifice coffee with a friend. But then the day will come when you know that you can handle a lower grade in exchange for relationships. It's a give and take, one that you will learn as you balance a complex, crazy life.

You're not a failure if you decide to miss your son's basketball game because you have to study. Guess what? One day you will graduate and have "RN" behind your name. You can show your son that pursuing your dreams is important.

You're not a failure if you decide to go to you sister's baby shower and forgo that study group this week. Guess what? One day you will graduate and have "RN" behind your name. You can show your sister that being there for her is important.

Give and take. It's a fact of life, and remains true even for nursing students. Give yourself some slack. Don't beat yourself up over every little decision you make, because one day you will look back on this time and see that it was through these fires of everyday trials that made you a better person. A better nurse. A better friend. A better spouse. A better parent. You can look the scared parents in the eye whose baby is in the NICU and be able to say with full confidence, "I will do everything I can to help your child." Why? Because it's the "right" thing to say? Or because you *know* what it's like to be placed in a situation that exposes your own anxiety, fear, sleeplessness, and desperation. In that moment, you can be glad you learned balance.

The Myth That You Can't Rest

By now you have figured out your study habits. You've heard it all. Everyone says you shouldn't study the day before a test. Everyone says you shouldn't save paperwork to the last minute. Everyone says Mental Health is the hardest class. No, everyone says Mother/Baby is. No...the list goes on. Everyone has an opinion about everything. Do this, don't do that.

You know what? There is one constant amidst all that.

You need rest.

You cannot escape sleep. It's an inevitability. The fact is, tired nurses are bad nurses. I'm not saying that every time you don't get rest equates to you making a

24

mistake and killing someone. What I am saying is that, eventually, you will be mean to someone. Lack of sleep produces irritable people. You'll snap at your coworker. You'll yell at your kids. You'll argue with the doctor. And yeah, you might make a mistake and harm a patient.

You Must Rejuvenate

Sleep is the main way this happens, of course. But there are other ways to replace the exhaustion of nursing school with fresh energy. What brings you rest? Is it reading? Getting away from the noise of your house for a few hours? Hanging out with friends to watch a movie? Crafting, gaming, or exercising?

Sleep, and do those things. Nurses are notorious for forgetting self-care. In fact, if there is one thing to take away from this guide, it should be that. Take care of yourself and you will be a better person. Period. Not just a better nurse, although that's true, too.

I was in one of those middle semesters when the opportunity came for me to go to Bolivia for a medical missions outreach. One of the reasons I pursued nursing was to travel and serve needy people. Yet the Bolivia opportunity made me wrestle with the decision. It would mean missing almost two weeks of school, spending a lot of money, and perhaps hurting my grades. But I decided to go, and you know what? It was the most fun, relaxing thing I've ever done. I know that hiking the mountains of

Bolivia carrying medical supplies, tents, and personal belongings isn't most people's idea of rest. But for me it was. We saw over a thousand patients in ten days. We helped orphanages, schools, churches…some people walked miles and miles just to see a doctor. Some were receiving medical care for the first time in their lives.

When I returned stateside I was rested and rejuvenated, ready to tackle my final semesters. I had some catching up to do, of course. But it was worth it, because part of going was taking care of myself, investing in my passion, and being reminded that there is life outside of school.

Chapter 4 – Nearing Graduation

One of the things that struck me as I gazed out at my classmates one morning was that this was a collective accomplishment. Graduation isn't a personal thing. It involves everyone in your life. We had achieved this *together.* There were days I didn't think I would make it to the final semester, but it was my friends, family, and classmates that helped me get there. And of course, my amazing instructors and professors. I had worked as a tech, still managed to be involved in community and world outreach, gotten relatively good grades, and met an awesome guy I thought I might like to be in relationship with when I was through.

It's a big deal, my friends. Don't let anyone tell you anything different.

The Myth that Graduating Isn't All That Hard

We all have those people in our lives. The ones that don't understand, and try to tell you that it doesn't take much to go to class and get a diploma. Thousands of people do it every day. And really, how hard is it to roll out of bed, go listen to a professor drone on and on about diabetes and Protonix and cirrhosis, and that other disease you can never remember? What was it again?

Maybe you believed them before you started. Maybe getting your pre-reqs wasn't all that hard for you. Then you walked in to your first test, looked it over and had no idea what half the words even meant.

I have some choice words for those people who say that nursing school can't be all the difficult. But for now, I'll just say this: don't listen to them.

Graduating Nursing School is a Huge Accomplishment

You should be darn proud of yourself. Your family should, your friends should, your neighbor should...everyone. Because nursing school is unique. There is no right answer on a test. They are *all* a good answer, you just have to choose the *best* one. Try telling that to a college algebra professor. They will look at you like you have three heads.

Not only are you in class for eight to twelve hours a week, but you are also in clinicals for ten to fourteen hours a week. To be honest, no one else will really understand except other nursing students and RN's. But that's okay.

I know you. I know the hard work. I know the tears. I know the exhaustion. My friend, I promise it will

28

be worth it. So go to your pinning ceremony with pride. Invite everyone. Sit with your classmates and feel good about yourself.

The Myth That After Graduation The Real Work Begins

Maybe there is a rumor going around that graduation is a breeze compared to what comes next. NCLEX. Job hunting. Getting back to real life. Making friends again. While there is a little bit of truth to that, let me just nip that in the bud. Right now.

Make Connections

Trust me. Getting through graduation is ten times harder than passing the NCLEX. You might study for a couple months and then take the test. But to graduate, you invested two to four years of your life. And let me say this with as much force as possible: promise me, PROMISE ME, that you will network in these last days. To be honest, you should have been networking the entire time. This is the fatal mistake I made. I didn't put myself out there enough. I have a more laid back type of personality (you have probably figured that out already.) I figured that with a little work the jobs would be there.
They weren't.

Guess who got hired first? The networkers. They were making themselves indispensable to the nurses on the unit. They introduced themselves to the managers. They made friends with the techs and secretaries. They happily bathed patients even though what they wanted to be doing was starting IV's and watching surgeries.

This is harder than the NCLEX. Take my word for it.

I didn't get hired in the ER I worked at as a senior nurse tech because I never bothered to meet the managers. The nurses and patients loved me, but the manager had no idea who I was.

I didn't get hired on the med/surg unit I was a tech on because I didn't let the manager know I wanted to work there as an RN. When I finally told her, she had already filled the postings with others. I was a good worker, I just was too quiet. I came, did my job, and went home. I didn't network.

I know you're thinking, "Wow, she's being repetitive on this networking thing." You're right, I am. But let me be honest with you. You won't get the jobs you want if you don't look people in the eye and talk to them. You won't get the jobs you want if you don't step out of whatever protective comfort zones you've built around yourself to keep from being rejected. You won't get the jobs you want if you assume you're so awesome managers will stand in line to hire you.And you won't get the jobs you want if you rely simply on your work ethic in the classroom and in front of the preceptors and managers.

You will more likely get the jobs you want when you take as much initiative in relationships with decision-makers as you do with studying for tests.

So take it from me: accept the fact that nursing school isn't just about academics. It's about developing a well-rounded skill set that includes growth in areas that have absolutely nothing to do with grades.

Chapter 5 – Bonus Content

This chapter is broken down into three parts. The assumption is that you have graduated, and are now studying for the NCLEX. Again, the rumor mill is churning. This person took the test and got 75 questions. They failed. This person took the test and got 84 questions. They passed. On and on it goes, while everyone tries to figure out the secret to cracking the NCLEX code and passing.

The Myth That You Can Pass the NCLEX If You Do XYZ

I'll only say this once. Study for the NCLEX like you studied for all your other tests. That formula got you to graduation, right? Then don't change it. One trick, however, is this: if at all possible, take the NCLEX six to ten weeks after graduation. Two of those weeks should be spent resting, doing some fun stuff or getting caught up with people you've missed. Then, hit the ground running for those last four to six weeks. Study like you have never studied before. I give you full permission to hide in a cave.

Some resources that helped me were pretty much all the famous NCLEX study guides. Kaplan's, Lippincotts, the whole gamut. Get them all. Do them all. Do practice questions over and over and over again.

I went into the testing center just as nervous as I had been that first day on the unit. All the same emotions: terror, nervousness, anxiety. I wanted to throw up. I wanted to be strangled. I wanted to pass so bad, because I thought if I didn't, I would be a failure. I'd be one of "those" people who had to take the test twice. Guess what? If you pass on your second or third try, you still get "RN" behind your name. And someone interviewing you won't ask how many times it took you. A doctor is still a doctor if they get the lowest grade in the class or the highest grade in the class. A nurse is still a nurse if they passed with 75 questions the first try, or 240 questions the third try.

I got 240 questions. Half-way through my eyes glazed over. I left convinced I had failed.

Two days later, I sent my sister and mother into the bedroom while I waited outside. I made them check to see if I had passed or not because I couldn't do it myself. I literally couldn't. It was the longest two minutes of my life.

They came out dancing. That memory is etched in my mind forever. And it will happen for you too.

The Myth That Jobs Are Easy To Get Because There Is a Nursing Shortage

Let's just say this myth might be the worst of them all. It took me eight months to get a job. Like I've said, this was because I didn't network. (Have I mentioned yet the importance of networking?) But the delay was also because getting hired as a GN is just plain hard. Everyone wants nurses with experience.

So let me tell you this now. More than likely, you will not get hired at your first choice. It is next to impossible to get hired as a new nurse into the ER, OR, ICU, Pediatrics, L&D, and a host of other specialty units. Apply *everywhere*. And I mean *everywhere*. Every hospital within a thirty mile radius. Consider options like nursing homes. The reality is that the best experience you can get will be on a med/surg unit.

After waiting and waiting, going to a million interviews within my city and outside of it, I got a call one morning. My brother worked for an IT company that had the contract for a local orthopedic clinic. They were using contract nurses and one had called out sick. My brother had mentioned I was a nurse, so they asked him to call me. It was 0800 and I needed to be there ASAP. Could I fill in?

Absolutely! I rushed around like a maniac and pulled in at 0845. It was for an outpatient surgical facility working with a pain management doctor doing epidural steroid injections. Not my first choice by a long shot.

I had no idea what I was doing. The only question they wanted to know was if I knew how to start IV's. I of

35

course said yes, but I hadn't done any in 8 months (I didn't tell them that, of course.) I walked in as the doctor was doing his first procedure. I was told another patient was waiting, and I was to start a 20 gauge IV so they could get a small dose of anesthesia before the procedure.

Talk about anxiety. What if I couldn't start it? Then the anesthesiologist would have to start them all, and I would look like a complete failure at my first real opportunity.

I sat before the patient, acting like I knew exactly what I was doing. I talked to them the whole time. I don't remember a word I said, only that *pop*. I got it in the first try. Talk about a confidence booster.

From that point I was The IV Queen. Every job I've had I was always asked to start the hard sticks. And I was offered a job. Was pain management my passion? No, but to my surprise I loved my job. To this day the doctor is my friend and we will randomly send texts back and forth about silly things, even though we haven't worked together in years. My next job was med/surg at a large hospital. And you guessed it. I loved it.

Don't scoff at med/surg. It will teach you a host of skills, and you might actually find that you enjoy it. I was a preceptor six months in, a relief charge a year in, as well as an assistant Educator. I sat in on interviews. I taught new nurses all the time. I grew in confidence, got a unit award for leadership, and loved every second of my job. Well. Not every second. But most of those seconds.

The Myth That New Nurses Can't Kick Butt

I know this because I did. I'm not trying to toot my own horn. I was laid back, yes. But I was also full of confidence. Remember the humility we talked about? You can be humble yet still believe you're one incredible nurse. It's possible to be new at your job, still learning and growing, yet being good at what you do. It doesn't take much.

Are you compassionate?

Are you teachable?

Are you willing to try new things?

Do you like people? (This one is important. If you don't like people, you should probably choose another profession.)

Are you okay with asking questions?

Then you've got this in the bag.

As a preceptor, it was clear to me who had the skills and personality to do the job and who didn't. With a little bit of confidence, stirred with some humility and a dash of compassion, you'll do just fine. So go out there and change the world.

One Last Thing

Sorry. You thought I was done, but there's one last thing that is very, very important.

37

It is okay if you can't do this.

Nursing school, and being an RN, is not for everyone. Look. We all know that if you drop out you will *feel* like a failure. But I want you to understand this. You are not. Sometimes it takes more strength to realize our limitations than it does to just push through and ignore the voice that is saying, "This isn't the right path for you."

You will begin to notice something the further you get in. For some nurses, it is a calling. This isn't just a job to them. They love what they do because they were meant to be a nurse.

But there are also some nurses who choose this profession because it's a job and a way to get a paycheck. A job that is needed in every large city and small town. As long as there are people, there will be illnesses and accidents. Don't push yourself through school to come to realize you are this person. You won't thrive. You will be unhappy. Your coworkers will resent you. Your boss will dread when you are on shift.

Wouldn't it be better to realize this isn't a calling and stop? There is something out there for you, and it's okay if nursing isn't it. You have worth. You have dignity. Find what gives you those things, and don't force yourself to finish something just because you started it and don't want to appear weak or a failure.

One Last, Last Thing

I promise I'm done after this. Really. This time I'm done.

I knew I was where I was supposed to be when one day a doctor told me to discharge a patient and I refused. Now, generally this is a bad idea. 99.9% of the time you are to obey doctor's orders.

The patient was homeless. Her H&H was incredibly low. She needed a blood transfusion, and my suspicion is that the doctor wanted to discharge her because she wouldn't be able to pay for her stay or for any treatment. He probably hadn't looked closely at her labs, instead trying to free up the bed. I called hematology and they gave orders for a blood transfusion, and she had to stay the night.

The hospitalist was (understandably) upset. I argued with him for twenty minutes on the phone outside the patient's room, trying to explain what I had caught. When he finally calmed down enough for me to tell him he had missed the low H&H, the silence on the other end lasted five whole seconds.

"Ok, fine. She can stay." Click. No thank you. No, "Wow, Janelle, you just saved my butt."

My manager came over as I leaned against the wall. It was two hours past shift change. She put an arm around me. "You should have discharged the patient. And you shouldn't have, too. Well done."

I went into the patient's room. Her eyes were full of tears. I hadn't realized she overheard my side of the conversation. She listened as I advocated for her, not caring what her socioeconomic status was. Not caring that the hospital was busy and someone needed the bed.

She was a person. She was my patient. And she was the reason I knew I was doing what I was called to do.

You will have that moment too. Whenever it happens, sit back and smile. The rigors of nursing school will one day be worth it.

Love reading? Check out my epic fantasy series. Available in Kindle Unlimited, eBook, and print. Look for Part 2, *Rise of the Warlock King,* available in May 2018.

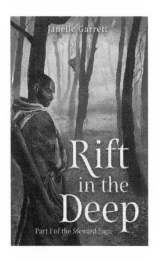

Sign up to my mailing list to receive a Steward Saga prequel novella for free, including staying up to date on my new releases, specials, and promos. One of my favorite things is finding awesome new work for my readers to enjoy.

About the Author

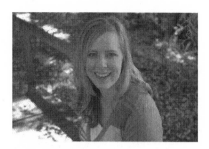

Janelle Garrett is a jack of all trades. Registered nurse, stay at home mom, medical records consultant...and writer. You can catch her on twitter @JanelleGwriter or at her blog, www.janellegarrettwriter.com where she tweets and writes about indie authoring, promoting other's works, and generally anything that she finds interesting...like religion and politics.

Made in the USA
Columbia, SC
30 April 2020

95118903R00036